Armchair Exercises
for
Fitness Phobics

Also by Susan Hooker.

Caring for Elderly People.
Understanding and Practical Help.

Recover Quickly
from injuries and other painful conditions.

Armchair Exercises
for
Fitness Phobics

Everyday Maintenance for the Busy,
Tired, Elderly, Infirm
and Straightforward Lazy.

By Sue Hooker.

M.C.S.P., S.R.P., M.B.Ac.C.

Illustrated by Maggie Humphry.

Email Sue at – armchair@suehooker.com
Sue's website – www.suehooker.com
Maggie's website – www.maggie-humphry.co.uk

Illustrations copyright Maggie Humphry 2006.

Note for Librarians: A cataloguing record for this book is available from Library and Archives Canada at www.collectionscanada.ca/amicus/index-e.html
ISBN 1-4251-0658-7

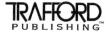

Offices in Canada, USA, Ireland and UK

Book sales for North America and international:
Trafford Publishing, 6E–2333 Government St.,
Victoria, BC V8T 4P4 CANADA
phone 250 383 6864 (toll-free 1 888 232 4444)
fax 250 383 6804; email to orders@trafford.com
Book sales in Europe:
Trafford Publishing (UK) Limited, 9 Park End Street, 2nd Floor
Oxford, UK OX1 1HH UNITED KINGDOM
phone +44 (0)1865 722 113 (local rate 0845 230 9601)
facsimile +44 (0)1865 722 868; info.uk@trafford.com
Order online at:
trafford.com/06-2416

10 9 8 7 6 5 4 3 2

Acknowledgements.

Special thanks to Emily for starting me off by putting the manuscript on to a disc for her technophobic mother, and for her continuing support. Also to Joe, whose patience and particular teaching skills have helped me so much.

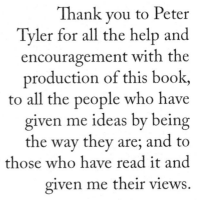

Thank you to Peter Tyler for all the help and encouragement with the production of this book, to all the people who have given me ideas by being the way they are; and to those who have read it and given me their views.

Maggie Humphry was like 'patience on a monument' while I sat beside her asking her to make changes to cartoons over and over again.

Thank you, Maggie, for your excellent contribution.

Foreword

Exercise makes you feel satisfyingly self-righteous; it improves your sense of wellbeing and increases motivation. It doesn't cost anything; but leotards, designer t-shirts, trainers and gyms do. And think of the time it takes.

This book is designed to increase mobility and help you to become generally healthier and happier.

It does not describe the type of exercise that improves heart rate or prevents heart attacks; but if you feel the urge to do more there is plenty that can easily be done without going mad, such as swimming and walking in particular.

Some exercises are included in more than one place. This is to maintain the continuity of the section with out having to keep referring back.

Depending on which category of the subtitle you subscribe to, you can adjust the suggestions in this book to suit your needs.

Why do I yield to these suggestions
Whose horrid images do unfix my hair
And make my seated heart knock at my ribs?

Shakespeare

This book is dedicated to all those people who do what I say and not what I do.

Please note.

No liability can be taken for people who fall over, strain, drown or in any way damage themselves while following the suggestions in this book.

The author presumes that readers are intelligent people who will use their common sense to use this book constructively and sensibly.

It is not designed as a book of treatments. People with specific conditions or who are worried by pain should seek advice from a physiotherapist, osteopath, chiropractor or doctor.

Read through each section before doing any of the exercises.

Contents.

Truth is never pure, and rarely simple.
Oscar Wilde

Much is to be endured.
Samuel Johnson

Interviewer: "What do you do to relax?"
Yul Bryner: "Relax! If I relaxed any more I'd fall over."

1 - Fitness Groups

The Fitness Phobics, the Fitness Freaks, the Wish they Coulds and the Think they Can'ts.

The **Fitness Phobics** sit at home in front of the computer or the television; or with their elbows on the table reading the paper. They may make the trip from their front door to their car to go to work, and down the road to the pub or shop.

Their conscience bothers them a bit. They worry about their backsides and their paunches. The articles on cellulite, blood pressure and cholesterol jump out at them from every newspaper and magazine they read.

**I sat and thought of exercise,
and then I stopped.
It's just not wise.**

Denham Tyler.

The **Fitness Freaks** wear shorts and expensive trainers. They pedal, row and pump two or three times a week. They give up hours of time to the God of Fitness, making the Fitness Phobics feel tired, just watching them.

They run in their lunch hour. Come rain, hail or shine they can be seen pounding the roads so they can take part in the next marathon, and become a respectable nine hundred and sixty sixth with their knees buckling and their faces grey with exhaustion.

The **Wish they Coulds** overlap with the previous group but are genuinely held back by their physical condition. They may be in hospital or have had some injury that prevents activity either temporarily or on a longer term basis. They may be 'getting on' a bit and becoming slower.

Not that actual age has got much to with anything.

"**Doctor, I've got a pain in my knee.**"
"**Don't worry, its old age.**"
"**Well, the other one's just as old and that doesn't hurt.**"

Others in this group may be disabled or find it hard to get around. But there are lots of things they can do, and many of them don't want to go to the gym much anyway.

The **Think they Can'ts** are people who have old injuries, chronic illness or pain, and have lost the confidence to push themselves a little. Some are nearing the top of the hill and think they are getting old; even if they are not.

Said the Table to the Chair,
"You can hardly be aware
How I suffer from the heat,
And from chilblains on my feet!
If we took a little walk,
We might have a little talk!
Pray let us take the air!"
Said the Table to the Chair.

Said the Chair unto the Table,
"Now you know we are not able!
How foolishly you talk,
When you know we cannot walk!"
Said the table with a sigh,
"It can do no harm to try;
I've as many legs as you,
Why can't we walk on two?"

So they both went slowly down,
And walked about the town
With a cheerful bumpy sound,
As they toddled round and round.
And everybody cried,
"See! The Table and the Chair
"Have come out to take the air"

Edward Lear

Which category are you?

After a few minutes each day spent stretching, moving, and breathing deeply the results can be very encouraging. You will be surprised at how quickly tight muscles relax and stiff joints become looser and with a smidgen more oxygen your brain moves up a gear.

These suggestions are remarkably effective and easy to incorporate into everyday life.

This book will help you feel happier with yourself without actually having to work too hard at it. It will help you to move about more freely, jump out of a chair, run up the stairs and turn your head round when you back the car.

Actually, it is a fact that exercise improves the auto-immune system. Also, it is proven that exercise increases endomorphines (natural pain and stress relievers) in the brain giving you a feeling of self righteousness and well being.

But BEWARE!

Exercise gets you hooked, so be aware of being too energetic or too disciplined, or it will not be long before a niggling enthusiasm has you signing up at the local gym.

2 - Fundamentals - Simple Truths

First - Stand Up! Stand Up!

**Peter White will ne'er go right.
Would you know the reason why?
He follows his nose where'er he goes
And that stands all awry.**

Nursery Rhyme

You are standing upright and balanced when a plumb line held by your ear falls past your shoulder and hip, and just in front of your ankle.

Nobody can function properly with their chin leading the way, their back rounded or their bottom sticking out. If you are leaning slightly forward all the time, gravity is pulling you down and making all your muscles work much harder to stop you falling on your face.

The natural curves of the spine should be maintained as far as possible whether you are sitting, standing or lying. If they are not, some muscles become too short, others too long; and the rather precarious upright stance we have adopted becomes threatened.

The most common fault is general sagging, with rounded shoulders and a poking chin. The upper thoracic spine also becomes too bent and you get a typical stoop. This sometimes shows as early as thirty or so.

It has the effect of drawing the back of your head down towards your shoulders thus shortening your neck muscles.

It creates an exaggerated curve in your neck which pinches the nerves to your arms.

Bad posture creates a knock on effect, which, as time passes creates more and more problems. It can cause neck and back pain, headache and Irritable Bowel Syndrome. Migraine, also, can be caused by faulty neck position. 'Tennis elbow', 'frozen shoulder', indigestion, palpitations, hip and knee pain, and sciatica; all can be influenced by the way you stand.

In most cases posture is easy to correct if you know what to do. It takes time and persistence, but it can be done.

He had been eight years upon a project for extracting sunbeams out of cucumbers, which were put into phials hermetically sealed, and let out to warm the air in inclement weather.

Jonathan Swift.

It won't take you eight years though; more like eight weeks, depending how much you practice. The trick is staying like that.

This is how you do it

- **Stand with your back and heels against a wall.**
- **Draw the base of your neck towards the wall keeping your face straight.**
- **Bring your head forward about an inch and you will be about right.**
- **Your low back should remain still, but with your bottom tucked in a little bit.**
- **Stretch up. Just lift your breast bone and stick your 'boobs' out a bit.**
- **Keep your knees straight.**

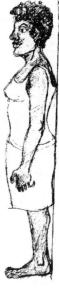

Now tall Agrippa lived close by,
so tall he almost touched the sky.

Heinrich Hoffman

That's all. The rest of you doesn't have to move.

- **Don't stick your chin up, if anything, tuck it in a bit.**
- **Don't breathe in hugely.**
- **Don't yank your shoulders back.**
- **Don't put your nose in the air or nobody will talk to you.**

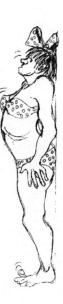

Look at little Johnny there,
Little Johnny head in air.

Heinrich Hoffman

In your brain there is a *postural centre* that tells you what position you are in. You try and alter the way you stand or sit but as soon as your mind isn't on the job your brain says "I don't recognize this" and puts you back how you were.

Therefore you have to train your brain as if it was a dog.

Do it again and again and tell yourself how much taller and better you feel. Gradually, it and you will do it naturally.

"You are old Father William," the young man said,
"And your hair has become very white;
"And yet you incessantly stand on your head
"Do you think at your age it is right?"

"In my youth," Father William replied to his son,
"I feared it might injure the brain.
"But now I am perfectly sure I have none,
"Why I do it again and again."

Lewis Carroll

When you are doing things that require you to bend, crouch, twist or hold an awkward position for a while, make a point of standing up straight and stretching yourself upright every now and again. It is very easy to get absorbed and spend far too long in one position, and end up crocked as a result.

Just Standing.

If you find yourself waiting for someone or standing in a queue it passes the time to be doing something useful.

- **Make sure you are standing up straight.**
- **Brace your knees back hard several times.**
- **Tighten and relax your bum. No one will notice unless your clothes are very tight.**
- **Roll your ankles out and then in, keeping your knees straight.**
- **Move your weight from one foot to the other.**
- **Stand on one leg; discreetly.**
- **If you have to stand for any length of time, put your feet apart a bit wider than you would normally; and just let your knees bend slightly. It makes you much more stable and relaxes the bottom of your back. They don't call that position 'at ease' for nothing.**

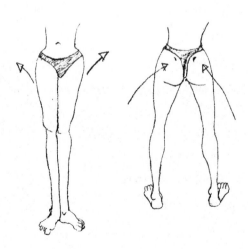

Second - Walk Tall

**"Will you walk a little faster" said the whiting to the snail,
"there's a porpoise right behind me and he's stepping on my tail"**

Lewis Carroll

Walking is just standing on the move. Fast walking is even better; it fuels your generator.

Make sure your feet face forward and you push off with the ball of each foot.

This action makes the calf muscles act as a pump and increases the circulation.

If you make an effort to step out you will maintain good movement in your hips. As you get older your joints get stiffer (unless you stop them) and there is a tendency to take smaller and smaller steps.

Walking up hill is especially good for the heart and lungs.

Stride along sometimes, swinging your backside from side to side.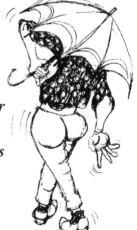

Don't lumber around.

Don't stick your feet out.

Don't bend forward from your hips or waist.

Look at your posture in shop windows and on CCTV screens.

Look at other peoples' posture.

Watch other people walk.

Sure, deck your limbs in pants,
Yours are the limbs my sweeting.
You look divine as you advance,
Have you seen yourself retreating?

Ogden Nash

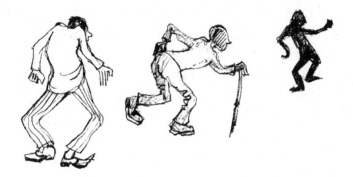

"It struck each man as he followed his neighbour
that the one before him walked very crookedly"

John Surtees

Try to incorporate this dynamic, upright new you into your everyday life.

Moving about at work.

Walking to the car or train.

Going up and down stairs.

Shopping.

In the house and garden.

Go for a walk specially to concentrate on your posture. Catch your shadow walking beside you in the morning or evening sun, it can be quite revealing.

Third - Sitting

"Sometimes I sits and thinks, and sometimes I just sits"

Anon

Many of us spend too many hours sitting due to the way we work; and partly due to changes in our modern life style. Some people sit down because they have to, following an accident or illness perhaps. Many people are confined to a hospital bed, sometimes for long periods.

Do you sit for long periods
in a car, van or truck,
in front of the tele,
in a plane or train,
at a desk,
in a chair?

For some people it is difficult to do much else, so this chapter is good for them.

Some people are just lazy or lack motivation to do anything else.

**The cure for this ill is not to sit still,
Or frowst with a book by the fire;
But to take a large hoe and a shovel also,
And dig till you gentle perspire.**

Rudyard Kipling

Whatever type of chair you sit in try to keep your back straight. Don't slump.

Use cushions or a pillow in your back if necessary. When you are relaxing you can lean back as far as you like, but still keep your spine straight.

Don't end up with your back bent like a hoop.

... stretched on the rack of a too easy chair.

Alexander Pope

If you are elderly, infirm or straight forward lazy; or if you are one of those people confined through illness or disability take particular note of the following.

If you sit leaning backwards all the time, your brain starts to think that position is upright. Therefore, when you stand up your brain feels as if you are leaning backwards.

This can be a cause of falls among people who are not very steady on their feet anyway.

Make sure you are sitting upright. Lean forward sometimes and put your elbows on your knees for a while. Look at *postural centre* on page 8.

Sitting at a Desk or Table

The chair should be of a height that your feet can be flat on the floor. If the chair is too high it makes you arch too much, and can cause backache. If you have short legs use a small stool, or the telephone directory, or something to put your feet on.

If the chair is too low, or you are too tall, you will slump forward to be able to see properly.

Put the chair close enough to the desk so that you don't have to lean forward. Sit close and upright with the weight going through your tail not your thighs and just tip your head down so you can see what you are doing. This applies to all types of close work.

Make sure your work is straight in front of you. Sitting for long periods with your neck on the skew is not good for it.

The desk or table should be of a height that you can reach the keyboard, book or whatever without having to lift your shoulders, or bend over to see what you're doing.

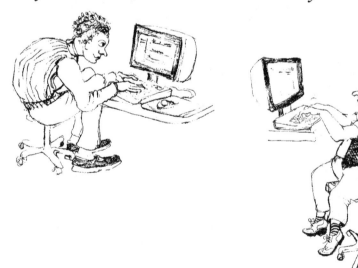

If you wear glasses position yourself so you don't have to tip your head back to see the book or screen. It can be a great source of headaches.

Many people have glasses specially for using with the computer but if you wear varifocals or bifocals try some 'Blutack' or chewing gum under the bridge to get them the right height.

Don't sit for too long. Many people sit for hours at a time absorbed in whatever they are doing. It addles your brain as well as stiffening your body.

Occasionally, sit up straight, circle your arms round and round and twist round both ways to look behind.

If you drive a tractor, forklift or some other agricultural or industrial machinery you will be spending a lot of time turning round, usually in one direction. Every now and then sit up straight and twist in the opposite direction. Get down and walk about a bit.

Walk around, stretch up tall and do some deep breathing to get your system working a bit.

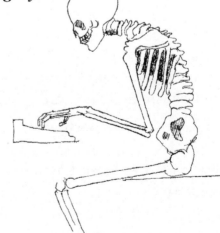

3 - The Exercises

**Now, here, you see, it takes all the running you can do,
to stay in the same place. If you want to get somewhere else,
you must run at least twice as fast as that.**

Lewis Carroll

This book is not for dogmatists and you are expected to use your common sense. Don't even try to do the things suggested if you know you won't be able to do them; or might damage yourself if you do. Take notice of changes in pains or discomforts and make decisions as to whether it is a pain that feels it is helping or pain that is causing damage.

Most people can tell the difference.

As a general rule some discomfort at the time is acceptable; however, if it continues when you stop or you are sore later that day or the next morning you have overdone it. Omit that exercise until the discomfort subsides and start again more gently.

Nothing you do should cause serious pain
either during or after doing exercises.

There is a condition called *Adverse Neural Tension* that is the cause of a lot of undiagnosed and persistent pain; therefore, I shall explain in more detail.

Inflammation in nerve roots near the spine will irritate all the muscles in the arm or leg supplied by them. The muscle spasm caused will clamp round the nerve preventing it from running freely.

This in turn pulls back on the nerve root in the spine.

Therefore, pain on some movements in the arm or leg may actually be the residual effect of damage nearer the spine. Stretching these parts too far will increase the inflammation in the nerves and muscles and make you worse. It is a fine line between helping and hindering, so think what you are doing.

If you have a pain and you don't know how you did it, it is probably from an old injury that is pulling somewhere or persistently bad posture.

There will be lots of exercises described. Go through them at leisure and then mix and match the ones that seem to help you and make you feel better.

If you get fed up with these exercises, make up your own. If something in your daily life is difficult, like putting your arm in your coat sleeve, for instance, turn it into an exercise.

Bearing in mind that this book is for the busy, tired, elderly, infirm and straightforward lazy, it is not *the number of exercises that is important; what is important is how you do them.*

It is only the effort beyond what you can do already that makes any significant difference. I know this goes against the philosophy of this book, but you have got to try a bit.

A few done carefully and thoughtfully once a day is better than half and hour going like a bull in a china shop. Although, due to the expected readership of this book the latter scenario is probably unlikely.

Bend a joint, and then bend it a bit more. Gently.

Stretch it as far as you comfortably can, then a bit more. Reach a bit further.

If a muscle is stretched slowly it will give, but if it is moved suddenly it will activate a 'stretch reflex' which will in turn make the muscle recoil and tighten.

Movements should be gentle and sustained, not sharp and jerky.

Muscles, ligaments or nerves that are over stretched can become sore.

This is particularly so when exercising your neck, shoulders and arms and your hips, lower back and legs. Look at *Adverse Neural Tension* on page 16.

If you were an athlete this would not be a problem. But anyone who has had sciatica, 'tennis elbow' or a painful shoulder does not want them again.

You could cheer things up a bit by putting on some music.

Stretch, move, dance around, jump up and down, or whatever you fancy.

If it feels good; do it.

Just move.

Do's and Dont's

Particular **Do's** include

Do think what you are doing.

Incorporate exercises into your everyday life.

If there is a movement you find difficult turn it into an exercise.

The benefit you get is proportional to the effort you put in (not the time spent).

Do what helps and don't bother with what does not.

Do it gently.

Do enjoy it: or at least pretend to, then you will.

Nobody can do it for you.

If it's tender rub it.

If it's stiff stretch it.

If it hurts be gentle.

If it helps do it again.

If it doesn't: leave it a day or two and try again more gently.

If one bit hurts: move everything else that doesn't hurt.

Make sure you can:

reach your feet, wipe your bum, scratch your back.

If you can't, do something about it.

Particular **Don'ts** include

Don't do neck movements if they make you giddy, cause pins and needles in your hands or upset your back.

Don't circle your head around. You can go forward and back, right and left and tip it sideways, but don't circle.

Don't sit with your legs straight out in front of you with your hips at right angles and your knees straight if you have back or sciatic problems.

Don't lift both legs off the floor at the same when lying. (Or when standing.)

Anywhere Exercises

Breathing

And now I see with eye serene
The very pulse of the machine;
A being breathing thoughtful breath,
A traveller between life and death.

William Wordsworth

Food, water and air are what keep you on the road.

Deep breathing increases oxygen to your head and whole body.

It keeps your brain working efficiently and body looking young.

It helps varicose veins by pumping the blood up from your legs by a suction action of the diaphragm.

It pumps the blood round and round generally.

It warms your feet up.

You breathe with three areas of your chest; top, sides and bottom, so you need to be in a position in which your ribs and stomach are not constricted. Sit upright in a chair or car seat, lie in bed with your knees bent, or stand up straight.

This is what you do.

- **As you breathe in stick your belly right out; like a small child's. At the same time, expand your ribs sideways and up and lift your breast bone up breathing in all the time.**
- **When you feel you are about to burst – sniff.**
- **As you breathe out pull your tummy in, squash your ribs down and push all the air out till you are like an empty paper bag – then huff.**

- **The more air you get out the more room you have for fresh oxygenated air to come in.**
- **Do that twice.**
- **Take a few normal breaths.**
- **In the middle of the next breath stop breathing.**
- **Hold your lungs full of air for as long as you can.**
- **Time yourself with the second hand on your watch. Gradually try to increase the time.**

Note.

This increases the oxygen absorption into the blood stream. It is particularly helpful for asthmatics and people with lung and heart conditions.

Fingers, Hands and Wrists

These movements are necessary to maintain dexterity and full use of the small movements of the hands and fingers.

- **Make a tight fist then stretch and splay out your fingers.**
- **Put your thumb across to your little finger.**
- **Bend each finger on it own. Keep the others straight.**
- **Keep your knuckles straight and bend your fingers only.**

This is very important for fine movements. You can't pick up small things if the end joint won't bend right down with the knuckle straight. These little joints are the first to get stiff as your hands become a bit arthriticy, which most peoples' do sooner or later depending on how hard they have had to work.

If the top joint won't go right down to touch to the to of the palm, give it a gentle push. Gradually persuade it to go a little further each time you try. Most joints tend to become stiffer over time if you don't stop them.

- **With your arm against your side turn your hand palm forward. Then with your fingers straight pull your wrist back and then forward. Twist your arm inwards so your palm is facing away from your side and repeat hand movements.**

- **Do the same again with your elbow bent and tucked in to your side. Move your wrist up and down with your palm up and then palm down.**

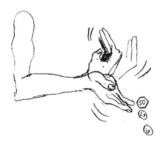 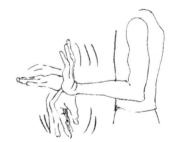

Faces, Grimaces.

"As a beauty I'm not a great star.
Others are handsomer far;
But my face- I don't mind it
Because I'm behind it;
It's the folk out in front that I jar."

Anthony Euwer

- **Move your jaw from side to side.**

- **Keeping your neck still, push your chin right out, then retract it, so it pulls the corners of your mouth down. Not a pretty sight.**

- **Pull the corners of your mouth apart in an inane grin.**

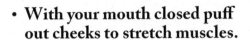

- **With your mouth closed puff out cheeks to stretch muscles.**

- **Raise your eyebrows; then** **scowl.**

- **Open your mouth wide; wider, to stretch the jaw muscles.**

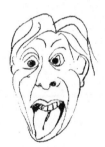

- **Make up your own faces.**

Note: These grimaces are good for headaches, neck ache, blocked sinuses and teeth grinding and sometimes dry mouth.

"Eye Eye"

> "You are old" said the youth, "One would hardly suppose
> That your eye was as steady as ever;
> Yet you balanced an eel on the end of your nose;
> What made you so awfully clever?"

Lewis Carroll

Your eyes are moved and focused by muscles. They need to be relaxed and fit like any others. Tense eye muscles cause blurring of vision because they don't co-ordinate or adjust to near and distance vision.

Note: If you do these exercises in public expect odd looks!

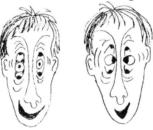

- **Look up and out and down and out as far as possible, keeping your head still.**
- **Look up and in and down and in.**
- **Put you finger one foot from your face and follow it with your eyes as you bring it towards your nose. In fact squinting. Stop when you see double. Gradually try to get your finger nearer your nose before going out of focus.**
- **Focus on a small object in the distance then on a small object close to you. And vice versa.**

Note: This is particularly important if you do close work or use a computer a lot.

Undercarriage

Pelvic Floor

This exercise is for men as well as women. It is generally uplifting.

The pelvic floor is a sheet of muscles across the bottom of your pelvis. It is these muscles that stop your insides dropping out. Necessarily there are various exits through it for babies and the removal of liquid and solid waste.

After childbirth and some gynaecological or prostate operations, they can become weak causing symptoms of prolapse, incontinence or sexual dysfunction.

You can do this exercise in any position any time.

- **All you do is 'pull up' the perineum (your 'undercarriage') as if you are trying to stop yourself wetting your pants.**
- **Hold it tight for as long as possible; then relax. Gradually try and increase the length of the time you 'hold it'.**
- **It is much better to do these exercises a few times several times a day than lots once a day. If you have problems such as leakage or stress incontinence, it may be a fairly long job and you will need to keep trying for several weeks to make a real difference.**

Note: If you have difficulties that worry you, you can often be treated by a specialist physiotherapist or nurse. Ask your Surgery Practice Nurse.

Bottom Half

Beauty for some provides escape,
Who gain a happiness in eyeing
The gorgeous buttocks of the ape
Or Autumn sunsets dying.

Aldous Huxley

- Tighten and relax your bottom. Really, really hard. (This may attract attention if done in public). This can be done in sitting or standing.
- Lift one side of your backside up and then the other, without rocking from side to side. You may have to stabilize yourself on the arms of the chair.
- Pull your feet up and down from the ankles and round and round in large circles.
- Keep your knees looking at the ceiling and turn your feet so that the soles face each other, then turn them out to look away from each other. This can be done in sitting or lying.
- Brace all the muscles in your legs, hard. Harder. Then let them relax.
- If you are going up or passing some stairs or steps, put the ball of your foot on the first one and press your heel down to give your calf a bit of a stretch. Gently if you have sciatica.
- Use the second stair to lunge forward to bend your hip and knee. (But not if you've had a joint replacement.)
- Keep the foot on the ground straight, and the knee straight.

Wake Up Call

> We climb out of bed with a frouzly head
> And a snarly-yarly voice.
> We shiver and scowl and we grunt and we growl
> At our bath and our boots and our toys.
>
> Rudyard Kipling

- Pinch all round the tip of your nose.
- Swirl your eyes round and round.

> See my lips tremble, and my eye-balls roll ...
>
> Alexander Pope

- With your nails, pinch your ears from the lobes up to the tips.
- Squeeze your ears in general.
- Put your fingers on your forehead and walk with your nails, from above your eyebrows up all the way up and over your scalp to the nape of your neck. If you bite your nails use a comb or something.
- Tighten each side of your bum alternately, as if you were walking fast.
- Brace your knees back and pull your feet up and down from your ankles.
- Take some deep breaths.

That should make you feel better.

Things to Do in Bed
(Respectable things)

Nobody can complain about exercises you don't even have to get out of bed for. If you do them before getting up you will be invigorated and ready to leap out of bed with enthusiasm. If you do them when you get into bed do them more gently and they will relax you and give you a good sleep. You don't have to do them all every time.

Less respectable things are also good exercise.

Feet and Ankles

She had very nice ankles and plenty of money

Daisy Ashford

- **Pull your feet up, and push down point your toes. Stretch hard.**
- **Circle your ankles round and round making as large a circle as possible. Keep your legs straight and still.**

Neck and Shoulders

- **With one thin pillow (more if you have to) roll your head from side to side as far as possible.**
- **Don't stick your chin in the air.**
- **Tip your head sideways on to your shoulder.**
- **Keeping your chin in, push your head back into the bed for a few seconds; then relax.**
- **Lift your head just off the bed a couple of inches and hold for a few seconds.**

- With your head straight, alternately circle the tips of your shoulders round and round. Forwards and backwards.
- Put your hands by your sides and roll the tips of your shoulders and your whole arms back. Roll your arms in so your hands face outwards.
- Pull your shoulder blades together; then stretch your arms across your chest to give yourself a big hug.

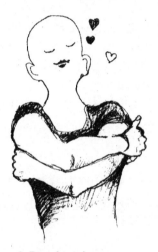

Knees, Hips and Backside

- Put your legs apart a bit. With your knees straight, roll both legs inwards so the big toes and knees face each other, then out away from each other.
- Bend your knees, keeping your feet on the bed; hollow the bottom of your back then flatten it down against the bed by tightening your stomach.
- Brace your knees straight back against the bed. Pull your toes up and tighten your thigh muscles as hard as you can, so they pull your kneecap up.

- **Do a few with each leg, keeping the knee absolutely locked straight. This is very important for knee injuries, arthritis and knee and hip replacements.**
- **Squeeze your buttocks together very tightly. Pull up 'undercarriage' muscles at the same time.**

Look at *Pelvic Floor*, page 25.

Do not do the next one if you have had a knee or hip replacement.

- **One leg at a time; bend one knee onto your chest and give a slow, gentle over pull with your hands. Keep the straight leg down flat with the back of the knee against the bed. Do the other leg. (If you have painful knees pull with your hands behind your lower thighs.)**

Now you will have to move a bit. Turn over onto your face. (For those beginning to summon up a bit of enthusiasm)

- **With your elbows bent put your hands flat on the bed under your shoulders.**
- **Lift your head and shoulders off the bed. Only lift the top half of your back; keep your belly button in contact with the bed.**

Do not do the next two if they cause back or leg pain.

- **Lean on your elbows and let your stomach sag on to the bed. Arch the whole length of your back. Just bending at the very bottom can strain the lower section and may create pain.**
- **Hold this position for fifteen seconds or so. Don't do it if it hurts.**

It is really better and easier if the next five are done on the floor; but if that is asking a bit much, the bed will do.

- Lying flat, face down. Keeping your knee straight; lift each leg up in the air alternately. Only move from the hip; don't arch your back or raise your pelvis off the floor. Put your hands under the front of your hips so you can feel if you take the weight off.
- Don't lift your pelvis off the bed or arch your back – that's cheating, and strains your back.
- Still flat on your face; bend one knee then lift it off the bed two or three inches, only moving your hip. Don't arch your back; this uses your backside muscles rather than the hamstrings.
- Do each leg alternately. Don't cheat by bending your hip and sticking your bum in the air. This good for saggy bottoms.
- Still lying flat; alternately bend each knee bringing your heel as near your buttock as possible.
- Don't stick your bum in the air. Put a hand under each hip so you can feel if you lift the weight off.

Roll back on to your back again. Put a cushion under your head.

- Bend your knees, feet flat on the bed, and with your hands on your thighs lift your head and run your hands up to your knees.
- Same as above but lift your right shoulder and arm towards your left knee and your left shoulder and arm towards to your right knee.

These are strong stomach exercises. Using the stomach muscles makes the opposite ones, that is, the back muscles relax.

These next ones are for fairly fit people.

DO NOT do them if you have had a hip or knee replacement. Be careful if your have a back problem.

- **Now sit up on the edge of the bed. (You could also do them on the sofa.)**
- **Put one foot on the top of the other knee, as if you were going to sit cross-legged. You can help it up with your hand if you need to.**
- **Use the opposite hand to support your foot, and put the other on your knee. Very gently put some pressure on the knee to stretch your hip. Stop if it hurts.**

Still sitting on the edge of the bed or sofa.

- **This time lift one foot up and put it on the bed beside you. It's difficult. Help it to get there by lifting your lower leg with your hand.**
- **Now put your hand on the outside of your knee and gently press it down towards the other one.**

This sounds more complicated than it is, but is a very good hip stretching movement. Stop if it hurts.

- **Lie spread- eagled for a few minutes, with your legs apart and your arms well away from your sides.**

See *Relaxation: Tension and Stress* on page 47.

Now you have to get up.

- **Sit up straight on the edge of the bed, put your arms out sideways and swing first one way then the other to look behind you. Not too violently. Mind your neck.**
- **Now stand up and windmill your arms round and round a few times in a relaxed fashion.**

And you are ready to be off.

Stirring Yourself in a Chair

These are good to do at the end of the working day, or if you can't get about.

- **Sit in an upright chair with arms, or a firm armchair with arms of a suitable height to rest your elbows on.**
- **You need to be upright so your head and neck are straight.**
- **Put your drink where you won't knock it over.**
- **Spend five minutes relaxing with your knees apart, and your hands on the arms of the chair.**

Then start.

See *Anywhere Exercises* on page 20.

- **Fingers, hands and wrists.**
- **Face and eyes.**
- **Neck.**
- **Pelvic floor muscles.**
- **'Bottom Half'**

You have hardly moved but already you will be feeling better. Now use a little effort.

- Sit up straight with your bottom right back in the chair. If the chair slopes back you may need a cushion behind your shoulder blade area.

- Press your elbows into the arms of the chair, or push up on your hands and let the waist area relax so that you exert some traction on your spine. Hold it a minute, go down slowly; and repeat it a few times.

- Repeat what you have just done, but while pushing up twist your rib cage from side to side. Next time while pushing up tuck your bottom in and stick it out; now wag your tail from side to side.

- Sit up with your back away from the back of the chair; put your right hand against the inside of your right knee.

- Twist to look over your left shoulder and gently push yourself a bit further. Repeat the other way.

- If you are on a kitchen type chair, hook the leading arm over the back as you twist and give an extra, very gentle stretch.

- Give yourself a big hug reaching your hands round to your shoulder blades. Bend forward and put one elbow on the opposite knee; then lift up and twist round to look over the other shoulder. Go both ways.

- Sitting straight, hollow and flatten your lower back.

Put your legs on a stool. (You may not be able to do this if you have a back or sciatic pain. Do *Things to do in Bed* instead. on page 28.)

- **Stretch your legs and feet out and splay your toes apart in a fan.**
- **With your foot pushed down from the ankle, point your toes down as hard as you can; tighten up the arch so you are pointing even more.**

This might cause cramp in the muscles on the soles of your feet. It's because they are weak. Keep practising and they'll be fine.

- **Brace your knees back really straight and with your feet pulled up to a right angle lift each leg, one at a time about one foot off the stool. Gradually increase the number of these.**
- **Squeeze your buttocks together really, really hard.**
- **With bare feet, slot the TV gadget between your big and second toes. Holding onto it tightly with your toes so it doesn't drop out, pull your foot up and down from your ankle. This exercise is very good for the arches of your feet. It will also change the programme if you don't concentrate.**

Take your legs off the stool

- **Sit away from the back of the chair or sofa; alternately circle your shoulders and stretch your arms out in front as if you were swimming the Channel. Reach out into the distance with each hand.**

The further off from England, the nearer 'tis to France -
Then turn not pale beloved snail, but come and join the dance.

Lewis Carroll

- **Now reverse the direction of your arms, and swim backwards, all the way home.**
- **Finally, sit up straight with your feet apart.**
- **Rock about, bend, stretch, twist, chuck yourself about like a rag doll; swing your arms around.**

Then sit back and relax.

Exercises in Standing

This is the time to put in a bit of effort in.

- **Stand up straight.**
- **Bend your head forward, tucking your chin in.**
- **Cave your chest in drawing the tips of your shoulders forwards to the middle of your front.**
- **Then gently start bending by rolling yourself forward.**
- **Pull your stomach in and only go as far as you can without bending your hips.**

This exercise puts the spinal cord on the stretch; therefore it must be done gently. If at any point you feel a pull down your back or the back of your legs: STOP. You can try again cautiously. If it becomes easier, go on doing it very gently. If it hurts, stop immediately.

See *Adverse Neural Tension* on age 16.

Arms and Shoulders

- **With your elbows bent, circle your arms round and round like a windmill or as if you were doing the front crawl. See *Stirring yourself in a Chair* page 33.**
- **Circle in the opposite direction; i.e. swim backwards, using overarm stroke.**

Do these next ones slowly, and cautiously. If they cause pain in your forearm go particularly gently.

- **One arm at a time, stretch up to the ceiling. At full stretch turn the whole arm inwards. Keeping it like that, move your wrist first forward and then back.**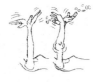
- **Then turn it out; bend your wrist forward and back.**
- **Stretch your arm out sideways at shoulder height. Twist the whole arm so your hand is palm up. Repeat the above wrist movements.**
- **Twist the arm right round the other way, as if taking a 'back hander'. Bend wrist again.**

See *Adverse Neural Tension* on page 16.

- **Put your right hand on your left shoulder. Try to reach round to the back of your neck. Put your left hand under the back of your right elbow, and gently pull your arm so your hand can reach further round. Keep your back straight while you do it.**

Neck

The head and neck should be in line with the body, not poked forward or leaning back against something. You can do them lying, sitting, or standing.

Do not circle your head. Stop if you are giddy.

- **Start with your head up and your neck straight.**
- **Turn to the left two inches; nod your head up and down a few times. Return to the straight position and repeat, turning the other way.**
- **Turn to the right as far as possible; now look up to the ceiling and down to the floor. Repeat, turning to the left.**
- **Facing forward bend your head from one side to the other. Ear to shoulder. Don't lift your shoulder.**
- **Facing forward tip your head forward and tuck your chin in. Pivot from just under your skull. Keep your back straight.**
- **Tip your head back pointing your chin up to the ceiling. If your head feels as if it might fall off cup your hand round the back of your neck to take the weight.**

Creaks and clicks are not important if they don't hurt. They will probably diminish if you stretch up taller.

Back

- Stretch one arm up to the ceiling. Put the fist of the other hand half way up your ribs.
- Bend sideways over your fist, without leaning forward as well. Keep the stretched arm really stretched. Go both ways.
- Holding on to something firm, swing each leg alternately forward and back. Make sure your body remains upright. Only move from your hip. Very clever people can do this without holding on.
- Swing your leg out sideways without rocking your body from side to side. Stay upright. Only move from your hip.

Go very gently with the next few stretches if you have sciatica. Stop if you create pain in your leg or back.

- To stretch the hamstrings (down the back of your thigh) put one foot well forward, and pull up your toes up from your ankle.
- Bend the back knee and stick your bottom out, keeping your back straight and your head up while keeping the front knee straight. You should be imitating a sweeping courtier's bow. Repeat with the other leg.
- To stretch your calf, go into a lunging position (as in fencing; with swords that is, not garden fencing), but keep both feet pointing forward, and the back knee straight with the heel firmly on the floor. Repeat with the other leg.

If you can; kneel on all fours.

Keep your shoulders and hips at right angles.

Humping and hollowing exercises.

• **Tuck your head in, to study your navel; tuck your bottom in, then hump your back up to the ceiling. Think of bringing your hips and shoulders nearer together by tightening your stomach.**

• **Now lift up your head, stick your bottom up and hollow your back, all the way up to your neck; bringing your stomach and chest as near the floor as possible. Feel each bit of your spine arch.**

Warning: Do not do this in front of the kids. It is very undignified.

Bobbing About in the Bath

Please read the instructions carefully. It is your own responsibility if you drown yourself.

Do not do those that require you to lie on your face.

Do not have the water too hot. It can make you very tired.

Do not do exercises in the bath if you would have trouble getting out again.

• **Fill the bath until the water is about level with your waist and have a bit of a soak.**
• **Do the *Things to Do in Bed* exercises for ankles, knees, hips, and pelvic floor (page 28).**

This is when you must be careful.

- **Lie on your back and slide down so your hair is under the water, but not your face.**
- **Stabilize yourself by pressing your head against one end of the bath and your feet against the other.**

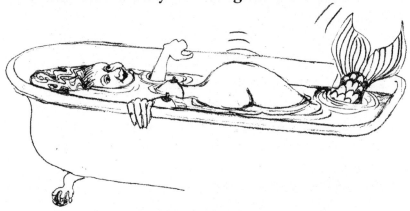

- **Lift your arms, and with your elbows bent, hold onto the edge of the bath with your hands.**
- **Keeping your hands still and your head still, slide and twist your backside from one side of the bath to the other. This will make your spine rotate from top to bottom and feels lovely.**
- **Still holding onto the sides of the bath, hollow your back, then flatten your spine against the bottom of the bath. Make each section of your back stretch. Start at the bottom and work up to your neck.**

The Power of the Shower

Some people hate showers. You have to stand up when you would rather lie down; and then get cold fiddling about getting dressed afterwards. But, there is the advantage of being able to run all that lovely hot water over your neck and down your back which is excellent for relaxing tired muscles at the end of the day. It's not as good as a soak in the bath though; but it is a good opportunity to loosen up and stretch the stiff parts of you.

You know which bits need attention so use exercises from other sections of the book that you know do you good or make up your own at the time.

Sitting on the Loo

- **Do all the exercises that can be done anywhere; hands, neck and specially eye and face contortions.**
- **Massage your thighs; at least, slop them about a bit. Go round and round with your knuckles, or your elbow.**
- **Do the backs and the fronts.**

This will help sciatica and painful knees.

- **Rub firmly in circles up the outsides, from knee to hip.**

Good for constipation and digestion in general.

- **Lift your heels off the floor alternately, to tighten your calf muscles.**
- **With your heels on the floor, lift your toes up.**
- **Put your feet apart and swing your knees together and apart as far as possible.**
- **Do arm swinging if there is room. Don't fall off the loo.**
- **Twist round to look at the wall behind you. Keep your bum still to avoid accidents.**
- **Put one foot onto the other knee and massage Arnica cream into it. This is a simple and effective way of helping sore or tired feet.**

Kitchen Sink Exercises

It starts when you sink in his arms:
And it ends with your arms in the sink.

Anon

- **Put on some cheery music.**
- **Jig about every now and then.**
- **At the sink or work surface stand with your feet apart; it relaxes your back.**
- **Swing your hips forward and back, and from side to side.**
- **Lift each heel off the ground alternately, in time to the music.**
- **Tighten your knees back; relax, and do it again. Don't stick your bum out.**
- **Stand up tall and straight every now and again. Put your hands in your back, a little bit higher than your waist, and arch back to have a good stretch.**
- **Do press ups against the work surface or sink. Stand about three feet away and lean forward to put your hands on the edge; bend your elbows so your chin goes towards the surface and then straighten your elbows to push you upright again.**
- **Squat, holding on to the sink and a chair; then tuck your bum in and stick it out; and shake it from side to side.**

Don't do this if you will be unable to get up again.

- **For the young and fit only; and certainly not if you have a back problem or a new joint.**
- **Hold on to a chair and swing one foot up on to the work surface, 'a la Can Can'. Both legs should be as straight as possible.**

Do one leg at a time.

Don't do it with a glass in your hand.

Some jobs can be done sitting down.

Peeling the 'veg', for instance.

Ironing: why can't you iron sitting down?

It's only a matter of lowering the board and getting a chair. In the Summer, use an extension lead and iron outside in the garden, or on the balcony.

Don't spend too long on the same job.

Move about in a purposeful fashion if there's room. Pottering about wears you out.

Passing the Time in the Car, Train, Truck or Plane

I suppose I should state the obvious and recommend that these exercises should be done with the car, truck or machine stationary. If you get stiff and tired and want to do yourself some good, I am sure you will have plenty of opportunity while waiting at lights or sitting in jams.

It's a good way of passing the time. You could even start a little class of fellow drivers on the hard shoulder which would pass twenty minutes or so. Maybe some of the Exercises that can be Done Anywhere and Standing Exercises would be suitable. If not, try these on your own.

Think whether you are all screwed up: relax.

- Hold the wheel where you are comfortable.
- Don't grip the wheel so tightly your knuckles go white.

Are your shoulders up under your ears?

- When stationary, put your hands on your knees, let your legs fall apart and let the tension go.
- Eyes get very tired driving so a few ogling exercises will relieve strain and make you safer.

See *"Eye Eye"* page 24.

- With your hands on the wheel, circle your shoulders in forward and backward directions.
- Wriggle your hands and wrists.
- Holding the wheel twist your body from one side to the other.
- Hollow and flatten your lower back against the seat. If your seat has an adjustable lumbar support it can be helpful to vary this from time to time on a long journey.
- Tighten and relax your backside muscles. Bop up and down; squeeze together and alternately.
- Pull your feet up and down and circle your ankles. Definitely only when stationary.
- Sitting up straight, turn to look behind you in both directions. Twist your body as well as your neck.
- If there is room straighten your knees and brace your thigh muscles strongly.
- Bend your knees and lift your feet off the floor alternately, to take the pressure off the back of your thighs a bit.

- **Breathing is very important; apart from keeping you alive, it keeps you awake and increases the circulation to your brain and legs.**

Do *Breathing* exercises on page 20.

This is very important on long and hot journeys; especially on motorways.

Open the Window (but not in the aeroplane).

At least in a train or plane all you have to worry about is what your fellow passengers think about your antics.

- **Do the relevant exercises from the section above.**
- **Move your feet up and down strongly to maintain the circulation in your legs.**
- **If you have short legs put something under your feet to take the pressure off the back of your thighs.**
- **Get up and walk about.**

4 - Relaxation

Tension and Stress

If you can keep your head when all about you
Are losing theirs and blaming it on you

Rudyard Kipling

Tension makes every bit of you work overtime. Stress causes tension but tension will also cause stress. Together they can cause actual muscle and joint disorders. No wonder stressed people feel so tired.

We are all programmed for a 'fight or flight' response when faced with stress. In these days of self control and so called civilized behaviour we don't fight when annoyed, usually, and we don't run away when frightened. The tension builds up in the muscles of the shoulders and arms which are prepared for fighting and in the backside and legs that are prepared for running away. This becomes a physical and mental habit and can create tension even when there is no stress.

There are people who feel that if they relax they are being lazy. We all need periods of rest. If you find sitting down difficult turn it into something positive. It will renew your energy levels; your immune system benefits from rest, and it helps recovery from illness or accident. You are not a machine; sitting down is good for you.

King Alfred did a great deal more than burn the cakes. His philosophy was to work for eight hours, sleep for eight hours and relax for eight hours. He still made time to set up the first judicial system; he laid the foundations of the Navy and he advocated education for everyone for starters.

Teaching your mind and body to relax is, again, like training the dog. Practise relaxing. Put it into your daily timetable; preferably at the same time each day so that your brain and body become trained to respond. Some people have difficulty getting into a routine because either they feel quite good and don't think they need to relax or they are so screwed up that they can't motivate themselves into doing it at all. Try to discipline yourself into going to lie down; say to yourself "I really need to do this," and it will gradually become a habit. Until you do relax you wont realise how tense you were.

If you want to do something, make a habit of it;
if you want not to do something refrain from doing it.

Epictetus, 1st-century philosopher

Practice it for about ten to fifteen minutes at least once, preferably twice every day. Remember what it feels like to be without physical or mental tension, so you can reproduce that feeling at other times. When you get good at it you will look forward to doing it and enjoy it.

Here in this little bay,
Full of tumultuous life and great repose,
Where twice a day,
The purposeless, glad ocean comes and goes.

Coventry Patmore

This is what you do.

Turn your phone off and make sure you are not going to be disturbed.

- **Lie flat on the bed with your arms and legs wide apart. With your arms spread out you can't hit anyone, and with your legs stretched out you can't run away, so the 'fight or flight' pattern is broken.**

- **Think about letting the tension 'go'; not about what you are going to do when you get up.**
- **Consciously start breathing fully; let your body sink into the bed with each outward breath. Breathing and tension are very closely linked.**
- **Breathe slowly using the phrases, 'my arms are heavy', and 'my legs are heavy'. Repeat them in your head each time you breathe out.**

Think about what you are doing to prevent your mind 'from chasing mice'. Concentrate on what you are saying and what you are feeling. It becomes self-hypnosis. The phrases become triggers that relax you automatically. When you lie on the bed and say 'My arms are heavy', they will just go heavy. An extra advantage to this is that eventually you will be able to use those phrases anywhere. However, they wont make you so relaxed that you fall off the chair.

The time it takes to acquire this skill will vary from person to person; depending on personality, the degree of stress and how regularly you practice.

You can practice sitting up in armchairs, car seats, cinemas and dentists' waiting rooms; in the garden, in a field, or on the loo. Gradually you will bring it into many aspects of your everyday life. Just say the words.

Take a two minute break:

- **Sit down.**
- **Put your knees and feet apart.**
- **Put your elbows on your knees.**
- **Put your face in your hands, fingers in your ears; close your eyes.**
- **Take deep breaths in with the back of your chest and long huffs out through your mouth. 'Let go'.**

Remember to remember to relax.

Practice remembering to remember to relax.

Where ever you are, whatever position you are in: 'let go' now.

Pre-empt stressful situations, however minor, and relax first.

Try to be aware of situations that get you screwed up and prepare yourself by 'letting go' before the event not after. If you miss the train, the car breaks down or somebody pulls out in front of you try to recognise that it is a stressful situation and do something about it then and there and not wait till much later when you are about to snap.

Relax now; not later, when it's more convenient.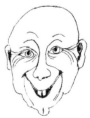

Relax your face.

Smile.

> The bough that's always bent will quickly break;
> But if unstrung will serve you at your need.
> So let the mind some relaxation take
> To come back to its task with fresher heed

Phaedrus, 1st-century poet

Many peoples' lives are so full and fraught that it is as if, like Gulliver, the Lilliputians have tied them down by dozens of strings. If they pull against them all at the same time, they can't possibly get up.

But, if they systematically remove one at a time, and put it aside; then, they will be free to move unhindered.

Spend some time of each session paying attention to your thoughts and worries. Each time you breathe out let another bit of you relax; and at the same time let one of your anxieties and thoughts go as well. Imagine them as kites or balloons that float off into the blue. Some from necessity have to be kept on a long string; but others can be cut and can sail away.

When we have a lot on our minds it is difficult to think about anything else. Make a little library in your head of completely unrelated and relaxing memories and thoughts, so when you need to get off the hamster wheel you have got something to pull off your mental shelf to think of instead.

Keep ahead of yourself and what you have to do, instead of constantly running to catch up. It may mean reorganizing yourself a bit, or even getting up earlier.

Finish today before starting tomorrow.
Then 'Take the new day by the forelock'.

5 - Massage

Everyone loves a massage; but not many people are lucky enough to be on the receiving end very often.

There are several ways of massaging yourself which will relax muscles and make the machinery generally run more smoothly.

Combine the massage of each area with exercises.

The general rule is to prod about in your muscles. If you find a bruised or sore area, get your fingers working at it. Feel for the tight bits.

Press into them quite deeply to stretch the muscle fibres.

Massage across them and around them.

Gentle smoothing with the flat of your hand will not help much.

General guidelines:

Do what feels nice.

Do a bit more on the tender areas.

Think what you are doing. Feel about.

Use enough pressure to do some good.

It is sometimes easier to press on the sore bit and move the part underneath. It's easier on the hands and less effort.

Don't work so hard that you cause pain. (You are trying to get rid of pain)

If you have a painful joint, massage the muscles above and below it. For example: if your knee hurts pay attention to the front and back of your thigh and the muscles of your calf. The tendons of all those muscles pass across the knee joint; therefore, if the muscles are tight they compress the inside of the joint. It is the same with the elbow and all the joints of the arms and legs.

Do what helps, and don't bother with what doesn't.

Ears.

**With monstrous head and sickening cry
And ears like errant wings.**

G.K.Chesterton

The body is mapped out on the ears in the same way as reflexology maps the hands and feet. By massaging your ears you can give yourself an all over once over with very little effort.

- **Using fingers and thumb work up from the lobe with gentle squeezing movements.**
- **Using your thumb and first finger nail pinch all over the ear including the inside bit. However, do not poke right inside your ear. Never put anything in your ear except your elbow.**

Face and Head

For headache, sinusitis, dry mouth.

When you're lying awake with a dismal headache,
and repose is tabooed by anxiety,
I conceive you may use any language
you choose to indulge in without impropriety.

W.S. Gilbert

Your face is one of the first places that tension, worry and pain show. Tight mouth and eyes and scowling brow are signs most people recognise. They can make you feel 'shut in' and even tenser. Headache and facial tension is often closely related to neck and back pain.

- **Sit back and relax for a minute. Shut your eyes and imagine massaging your brain with your finger; work all over it from front to back, from side to side or however you like.**
- **Massage all over your face and forehead with a round and round motion. Concentrate, particularly, from the corner of your jawline working upwards in front of your ears and up across your temple into the hairline.**

This area encompasses the muscles used in chewing; but particularly, in teeth clenching. If you grind your teeth, actually or metaphorically, this is for you.

- **Put the pads of your fingers on your skull behind your ears; rub round and round in small circles working up behind your ears to the top. Then do a bit on the muscles just above the ears.**

This is good also for tension and headaches.

This next bit is not for people with posh hairdos. Or people without hairdos at all.

Run your hands up through your hair; grab a handful and move your scalp round and round while pulling gently on the roots. Or you can hang on to your hair and move your head.

Move your hands a bit and repeat all over your head. It feels lovely.

Neck, Shoulder and Arm Massage

For headache, neck ache, chronic back ache, sinusitis, dry mouth, shoulder pain, tennis elbow and painful hands.

Neck

Keep your head up straight or rest it on the back of the chair; or do it in bed, with one pillow.

Don't do this with your head poking forward because it puts all the muscles you are trying to massage on the stretch.

- **Use the hand of the same side and circle your fingers up and down and round and round the side of your neck in small movements.**
- **Work all the way round under the base of your skull, from under your ears to the mid line at the back.**

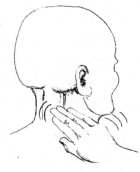

- Massage from the prominent bone behind your ear, down the muscle on the side of your neck, towards the knobbly end of your collar bone by your throat. This muscle sticks out if your turn your head. Make sure your head is upright and not poking forward.
- Put one hand behind the middle of your neck. Keep your thumb next to your index finger. Grab the muscles and give them a squeeze. Move your hand up and down the area squeezing as you go. Use the tips of your fingers to feel the hard, sore places; usually an inch or so out from the mid line. Go up and down. Use each hand to do the opposite side.
- Put a hand on each side of your neck. One hand circles up while the other circles down. Rub the whole area from under your chin and ears using your fingers to roll your head about in a relaxed circular fashion. Go round the back to the middle as well.

Shoulders.

Forty years on, growing older and older,
Shorter in wind, as in memory long,
Feeble of foot, and rheumatic of shoulder,
What will it help you that once you were young.

Harrow School Song

Hunched shoulders not only look ugly they cause headaches, sinusitis, dry mouth and low back ache.

- Grab the muscles on top of the opposite shoulder. Squeeze; move your hand up towards your neck then down towards the tip of your shoulder.
- With your fingers, knead the muscles in general; especially the knotty bits.

Arm Massage.

For neck ache, shoulder pain, tennis elbow, arthritic or stiff hands, painful fingers and thumbs, repetitive strain injury.

- **Pull and twist each finger and both thumbs. Not too hard.**

  What do you call a Judge without any fingers?
  See bottom of page.

- **With your middle finger and thumb pinch firmly between the bones of your forearm two fingers widths above the line of your wrist, move up and down an inch or two as well.**

- **Rub the front and back of your forearms. Use your fingers or knuckles.**

Massaging the front and back of your forearms helps in loosening stiff or sore fingers. The tendons you can see running across the back of your hands are the strings that work your fingers and thumbs. They are attached to the muscles of the back of your forearms. The front ones run across your palm in the same way.

- **Circle one wrist with the other thumb and middle finger and rub round and round working up your forearm; at the same time twist the forearm you are working on. Go right up to your elbow.**

- **Put one hand round the back of the upper arm on the other side; give it a good squeeze, and work up and down from the top to the elbow and back again. Don't miss the bit just above the 'funny' bone, it's often tight.**

Answer: Just'is Thumbs.

Low Back, Bum and Leg Massage.

For Sciatica, back pain and ache, stiff legs, sore feet; arthritic or injured knees and difficulty bending down. Bending down will be easier if your get your belly out of the way by pulling it in before you bend.

- **Roll each foot over a small bottle or foot massager.**

The sciatic nerve ends in the small muscles in the sole of the foot.

- **Sit sideways along the bed with one foot on the floor and one on the bed.**
- **Feel for the long, really tight bits in each side of the calf muscles. Use your fingers to work away at the knotty areas.**

You can also do this in your chair by half crossing one leg over the other and rubbing your calf up and down on the other knee.

The calves are sometimes very tender. It is important to loosen them up because they tend to hang on to the sciatic nerve and pull back up to the spine. Those people with acute back pain may not be able to do this; so ask someone to do it for you if you can.

In the same position rub each side of your Achilles tendon; above and behind your ankle bones. These muscles are very important for balance. *Balance and Preventing Falls* page 62.

- **Massage the muscle on the front of your lower leg.**

This muscle pulls your foot up. Giving it a good rub also helps digestion and loosens the bowels.

- **Still like that, knock the back of your thighs about.**
- **Just sitting, massage the front of each thigh using both hands. This can also be done on the loo.**

This is quite difficult. A wooden massager is quite helpful.

- **Have a go at your backside. Make a fist and work it round and round in the sore places. Or, when in bed put your fist under your bum and wiggle about on it.**

That's easier, as long as your don't have painful hands.

- **Put a tennis ball between you and the wall and do a belly dance; or a bum dance.**

> **Rubbing your backside**
> **each side of the crack**
> **will relax your neck**
> **as well as your back**
>
> Me

There is a reciprocal tightening between the muscles in that area of your bum and the muscles in your neck behind your ears. So rubbing your bum helps neck ache.

- **You can do this against the corner of a table or door frame. Wriggle your backside across the edge of the frame, working your way up and down by bending and straightening your knees.**

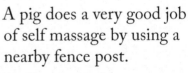

A pig does a very good job of self massage by using a nearby fence post.

It will amuse those around you anyway.

- Lie down on the floor with your knees bent. Spread your arms out to stabilize yourself.
- Swing your knees from one side to the other, massaging each cheek of your bottom against the ground.
- Sitting on a hard chair with arms; wiggle your bum in an indecent manner against the seat. As if you've got ants in your pants.
- With your hands on the arms, slide right to front of the seat and rub your bottom up and down across the edge. Don't slip off.

Feet.

Good for everything, but especially sore feet and chronic back ache.

- Sitting curled up on the sofa or chair; dig your nails into the soles of your feet. It feels lovely. Work, bit by bit over the whole of the bottom of each foot.
- Get hold of each toe, and give it a pull and a twist or two.
- Pull each one up as far as it will go to give it a good stretch.

Massage for General Circulation.
Do not do any of this section if you have cancer.

This massage will help with indigestion, constipation, tight chest and asthma, cold feet, and wonderful general relaxation. This massage is good to do lying down before going to sleep.

- **Using your fingers or knuckles; start at the tip of the opposite shoulder, massage round and round in small circles.**
- **Work along under your collarbone towards your breastbone, circling all the time.**
- **Go down the front of your chest where your ribs meet your breastbone.**
- **Change hands and massage round your ribs, from the middle outwards. Massage across them and around them.**
- **Repeat on the other side, any tender areas need doing a little bit more.**

The next part is for your digestion and bowels. See also *Bowels* page 73.

- **Using your right hand, start at the outer side under your right ribs. Work right across to the other side; using circular movements all the time. Change hands if necessary.**
- **Continue down the left side of your tummy to your groin, using your left hand.**

This is the direction the bowel runs. This circular massage helps release trapped wind and relaxes the bowel. So have pity on any other occupant of the bed.

- **With both hands go round and round about three inches each side of your belly button, then down the middle to the pubic bone.**

6 – Balance and Preventing Falls

**When sitting,
Just sit.
When standing,
Just stand,
Above all don't wobble.**

An old Chinese saying.

The muscles underneath the big part of the calf in your lower leg are responsible for balancing your leg on your foot; and therefore, your body on your leg, and your head on your body.

If these muscles are weak or out of balance it is difficult to stand on one leg long enough to put the other one forward when walking. This is particularly so if you walk slowly, as you have to balance for longer. Walking is like riding a bike; if you go faster you won't wobble so much.

The solution is simple; in theory anyway. (If you are elderly or infirm ask someone to stand beside you to begin with to give you confidence.)

Standing on one leg.

No holding on to anything – but be near enough to grab if necessary. To begin with you may only be able to do one second; but keep practising and you will get much better very quickly.

• **Then on the other leg.**
• **Practice.**

Try doing it every time you are waiting for the kettle to boil.

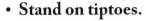

- **Stand on tiptoes.**

Hold on if you have to. Ten out of ten if you can balance like that without holding on. Twenty out of ten if you can do it on one foot.

- **Practice.**

For the really advanced balancer: walk on an imaginary straight line placing the heel of the leading foot against toe of the one behind; as if on the 'thin blue line'. Can you do it with your eyes shut?

Marching.

Note: This is good for balance, as well as physical and mental co-ordination.

- **March on the spot, lifting each knee as high as your waist – if possible. Don't worry if you can't get that high.**
- **More marching; more advanced. As your knee comes up clap your right hand onto your left knee, and your left hand onto your right knee. Alternately.**
- **More marching; even more advanced. As above only as your right hand claps on your left knee, put your left hand on your right shoulder, and vice versa. Some two-time music helps to keep you going.**

Many falls occur when changing direction in a hurry.

- **Practice walking and turning; walking and turning the other way.**
- **Walk; turn right around and walk back the other way.**
- **Lift your feet up as you turn; don't swivel. Don't go too fast.**

- **Turn in circles on the spot. Be very careful if your balance is unreliable.**
- **Walk on your heels.**
- **Walk on your toes.**

N.B. If your have problems with balance or unsteadiness make sure someone is close by to catch you if necessary.

7 - Getting About.

Crutches, Sticks, Scooters and Wheelchairs.

Crutches.

A significant number of people have to use crutches at some time or another. Sports injuries, falls and operations can all require a period of time using crutches.

The crutches or sticks must be the correct height. Just because you were given them in hospital doesn't necessarily mean they're right. If they are too high you can't push on them adequately and it scrunches your shoulders up; but if they are too short you have to lean forward all the time. Look at measuring for sticks but get someone to use a tape to get the distance from the floor to the hand grip right. If it's not right, adjust the height accordingly.

Suddenly not being able to get about is a great way to get fed up; and many people turn into couch potatoes. The muscles that are not being used get very weak, and the joints stiff; particularly if you are in plaster.

Although the plaster will inhibit movement, the muscles can still be worked by bracing them inside the plaster.

Tightening muscles around the fracture stimulates the growth of new bone and the fracture heals more easily. Start gently a week or so after the injury.

Move all the other parts of you, specially the joints above and below the plaster.

If you use your time well and follow my suggestions you will be up and running very much more quickly.

Sticks.

Many people feel unsafe when walking outside their house and worry about falling over. A stick just gives a bit of support and is a great way of beating a path through a crowd.

If you need one, try and find one of the new ones with a specially shaped hand piece. They are much easier to use and very much more comfortable. Mobility shops sell them. Some also have a 'thing' that will allow you to hang them on the back of chairs or whatever, rather than having them fall over whenever you put them anywhere.

Measuring for a stick.

If the stick is too short you have to bend.

If it is too long you get shoulder ache and it upsets your balance. You need to be able to press down on it.

- **Put your arm by your side with the elbow slightly bent; not too much, and your wrist pulled back; as if you were holding the stick.**

- **Get someone else to hold the stick upside down and measure to the base of your hand. Cut it off and make sure to put the rubber ferrule back on. It is dangerous to use a stick without one.**

CUT

Scooters and Wheelchairs.

I am in favour of using any prop, bike or trike that will help you get about; whatever your age.

Many people refuse to use these things for various reasons; often because they think it makes them look 'disabled', or they are 'giving in'.

In fact it gives you a new lease of life.

An ordinary wheelchair gives a freedom to two people. Instead of not going out, or having to go short distances at snails pace, two people can enjoy a jaunt together.

An electric scooter is even better. You don't have to live in it; it just gets you from place to place – fast. It can be parked outside the shops, pub or wherever, and in you go. They make double ones now too.

A letter in the newspaper complained about an elderly lady in a buggy flying down the middle of the pavement with mobile phone clamped to her ear. Old people these days!

Don't sit at home. Get out there: one way or another.

Gardening.

And if you voz to see my roziz
As is a boon to all men's noziz,-
You'd fall upon your back and scream-
'O Lawk! O crikey! It's a dream!

Edward Lear

Gardening jobs create good opportunities for keeping supple and doing yourself a bit of good while enjoying yourself.

Combine gardening with stretching, moving and striding about.

It's also a good way of ending up with back ache.

- **Do the weeding on your hands and knees.**

It is much better for stiff joints and sore backs than bending down.

- **If you think you will not be able to get up, have a stool nearby to help. You could even sit on the stool and weed between your feet.**
- **If you do bend down, bend your knees and put your feet well apart. You can rest one elbow on your knee to give some support if necessary.**
- **Whichever way you do it, don't tip your head back to see which bit you are going to do next; it is not good for your neck and can cause pain and headaches.**
- **Stretch your arms out to reach all round you.**
- **Sit back on your heels, if you can, and admire your work.**
- **Pruning is a good time to reach out in all directions.**
- **If you have a back or neck problem put pot plants on wheels.**

- **Change jobs often so joints and muscles don't get over tired from being in the same position for a long time.**
- **If you have room walk about your garden; you never know what might see.**

And spectral dance, before the dawn,
A hundred vicars on the lawn;
Curates, long dust, will come and go
On lissom, clerical, printless toe;
And oft between the boughs is seen
The sly shade of a Rural Dean.

Rupert Brooke

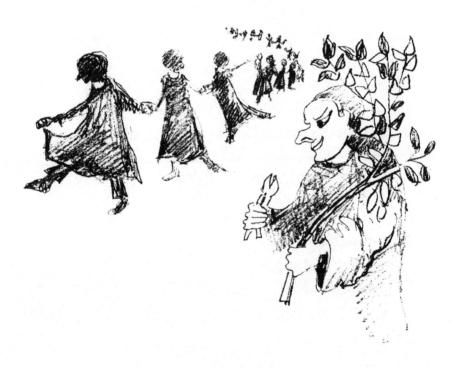

Eating.

*For my part I mind my belly very studiously and very carefully;
for I look upon it, that he who does not mind his belly,
will hardly mind anything else.*

Samuel Johnson

As there are nearly as many diets as there are people it seems sensible to take a middle line between what basic common sense tells us is right; and what you know makes you feel better, while avoiding foods that you know don't.

What the latest fad is or what recent research proves and then disproves is just a series of 'red herrings' to put us off our eggs.

The basic rules are:

- **Eat as many vegetables and fruits as you like.**
- **'Filling' in the form of brown bread, pasta, rice and porridge oats.**
- **Protein, for energy; such as fish, meat, peas and beans; as in baked, soya and chick peas.**
- **Lots of garlic.**
- **Lots of water.**
- **Less coffee and sugar**
- **Moderate alcohol.**

Apart from other things alcohol is a good muscle relaxant. Hence 'legless'.

*And Noah he often said to his wife when thy sat down to dine,
I don't care where the water goes if it doesn't get into the wine.*

G.K.Chesterton

Many people have intolerances to foods such as wheat, gluten and dairy products. This is too complicated a subject for this book, but, if you suspect food of some sort is upsetting the system, medical and/or complimentary help should be sought.

A good vitamin and mineral supplement is useful. An established make from a health shop will have the right combination of everything that is needed to be absorbed properly by the body, and then used fully. You tend to get what you pay for. It may turn your pee a wonderful golden yellow.

A good food table

Little	Normal	Lots
Animal fats Cheese	Fish, like whitebait & herrings	Cauliflower
		Sprouts
Coffee	Lamb's liver & kidney	Spinach
Tea Beer	Chicken not battery reared	Broccoli
		Beetroot
Sugar Cakes & biscuits	Oysters: good for prostates and sex life.	Carrots
		All vegetables.
Cream	All seafood	Salad
Pastry	Cottage cheese	Garlic
Fry ups	Live yoghurt	Olives
Salt	Brown rice	Avocados
	Pasta	Pineapple
	Lentils & beans	Apricots
	Potatoes especially new	Bananas
		Melons
	Brown bread	Prunes
	Dried fruit	Tomato
	Dark chocolate	Parsley
	Olive oil	Most herbs
	Nuts: not peanuts	Watercress
	Wine	Black pepper
	Guinness	Tomato paste
	Marmite	
	Ginger	
	Molasses	

If you are all over too fat, it would be wise to try and lose a bit.

Losing a little, helps a lot.

Every time you take a step you put four times your body weight through each knee at each step.

If you can lose 5lbs (11kg) there is 20lbs (44kg) not going through your knees. That's 4 bags of potatoes.

Every pound on your stomach puts 5lbs (11kg) through the bottom disc in your back. (Where your sciatic nerve originates).

If you have 'fat bits' but are not all over too heavy, exercising the muscles underneath helps. For example: stomach exercises for a paunch.

On the other hand the Greeks say, "a man without a paunch is like a house without a balcony".

'Tis not the eating, 'tis not the drinking that is to be blamed, but the excess.

John Seldon

Why Can't I Lose Weight? by Martin Budd N.D., D.O.

Published by Thorsons. ISBN 0-00-712065.

This book is very helpful for people who make a serious effort but never seem to get very far.

The Vitamin Bible by Earl Mindell.

Published by Arlington Books ISBN 0-85140-672-6.

An excellent, clear, easy to read guide.

Bowels.

If the bowels get chocked up, the system slows; you absorb more nutrients and fluid than you need and you put on weight. The stools get too dry and you become even more bunged up.

Constipation also has the effect of pushing back up and causing indigestion, wind and even palpitations. Breathing sometimes becomes shallow because there is no room for the lungs to expand downwards.

If food takes too long to go through it is possible to absorb toxins, which can cause numerous problems such as muscle stiffness, headache, nausea and food intolerances.

Getting the Bowel Moving.

Dear Doctor, I have read your play,
Which is a good one in its way,
Purges the eyes and moves the bowels,
And drenches handkerchiefs like towels.

Lord Byron

- **Drink water.**
- **Potters' Cleansing Herbs. (Health Shops)**
- **Prunes, figs etc. These can be bought in concentrated cubes.**
- **Curry helps to clear the chest, bowels and skin. They are all organs of elimination.**
- **Massage.** See page 52.
- **Exercise: the more energetic the better. Sorry. Walking is good too.**

Bowel diseases and Irritable Bowel Syndrome (IBS) often cause the bowel to be too loose.

Some cases of constipation and IBS may caused by a problem in the neck. There is the very important Vagus Nerve that affects most of the digestive system; indeed, all your innards that you are not aware of; pancreas, liver and gall bladder for instance. It passes from the base of the skull all the way down to the lower stomach area.

8 - Entertaining your Mind

Use it or lose it.

Your ability to concentrate, to reason, to visualise, to imagine, to make decisions, to solve problems and to think clearly and creatively depends greatly on how well and how often you exercise your mind.

Tom Wugek

Concentrate.

What are the feet of a centipede like?
Think about the social structure of a bee hive.
Think about The Universe.
The population of China.

Where does the sea come from?
How does the moon get up in the sky?

Joe, aged 4

- **Really study an object in the room for two minutes without letting your mind wonder onto other things. What shape is it? What is it used for? Where did it come from? What will happen to it when you don't want it any more? You can think of a lot of things in two minutes.**
- **Study something you can see out of the window.**
- **How many circles can you see around you.**

- **Sing.**
- **Recite poetry.**

- **Say good morning in as many different languages as you can.**

I said it in Hebrew- I said it in Dutch,
I said it in German and Greek;
But I wholly forgot (and it vexes me much)
That English is what you speak.

Lewis Carroll

Practice Imagining.

Smells: the sea, blossom, food, farts. What else? Smells can be very evocative and jog all sorts of memories.

Tastes: salt, shampoo, apricots. What else do you like or dislike.

Running: thumping along, puffing, flying.

Enjoying yourself: whatever turns you on.

Go on a jaunt: you can go anywhere you want.

Listen.

To the noises around you: people, birds, the wind, a train in the distance, your own breathing. Anything; but open your ears.

Listen to the quiet.

To other people speaking. What are they saying?

I said it very loud and clear,
I went and shouted in his ear.
But he was very stiff and proud
He said "You needn't shout so loud".

Lewis Carroll

Who Needs Habits?

Habits, mental and physical, enable us to get through life without having to think about it.

Here are some suggestions for altering habits:

- **See different people, if possible. It may take a bit of effort.**
- **Try talking to people you don't normally talk to. You may learn something and find yourself talking about subjects that are new to you.**

> "The time has come", the Walrus said,
> "To talk of many things:
> Of shoes and ships – and sealing wax –
> Of cabbages and kings-
> Of why the sea is boiling hot –
> And whether pigs have wings".
>
> Lewis Carroll

- **Wear different clothes. Change your hair. Alter your glasses.**

> I was thinking of a plan to dye
> one's whiskers green.
>
> Lewis Carroll

- **Change your routine. In fact, cancel routines.**
- **Don't do everything the same way everyday; think what you can change.**
- **Clean your teeth differently. Up and down, round and round; use the other hand. Start back to front.**
- **Watch different television programmes. They may be interesting, they may be irritating; they may make you laugh when you weren't expecting it.**

- Read a magazine or newspaper that is new to you. It may give you a different perspective, whether you agree with it or not.
- Read a book that is totally different from one you would normally choose.
- Try new foods. Most of us eat in a pretty repetitive and boring way.
- Brush your hair with the other hand. (Brushing your hair is very good for your health). But that's another subject.
- Turn the tap on with the other hand.
- Sit in another chair.
- Make a game of it all.

Keep Learning.

The best thing for being sad .... is to learn something.
That is the only thing that never fails.
You may grow old and trembling in your anatomies,
you may lie awake at night listening to the disorder of your veins,
you may miss your only love,
you may see the world about you devastated by evil lunatics,
or know your honour trampled in the sewers of baser minds.
There is only one thing for it then – to learn.
Learn why the world wags and what wags it.
This is the only thing which the mind can never exhaust, never alienate,
never be tortured by, never fear or distrust, never dream of regretting.

T. H. White

Start a course. What are you interested in that you would like to know about? It doesn't have to be high powered; it could be a weekly afternoon or evening class. As well as Local Authority classes, W.E.A. do day and evening classes all over the country on subjects of general interest. There are a lot of educational subjects on television too.

Learn a language.

Make up a limerick. A funny one.

Look up things .. ask yourself "I wonder what, or why".

Teachers open the door but you must enter yourself.

Chinese Proverb

Practice Remembering.

"The happiness (sic) of that moment," the King went on,
"I shall never forget it".
"You will, though," the Queen said,
"if you don't make a memorandum of it".

Lewis Carroll

Remember all the good things that happened today, however small.

What did you do yesterday? Did you enjoy it? What was the best thing.

What you were doing five years ago?

What is your earliest memory?

Who was your best friend at school? Do you know what they are doing now?

Name the characters in the last book you read. What did you like about it?

What did you buy last time you went shopping? Was it a waste of money or are you pleased with your purchase?

Remember telephone numbers instead of looking them up every time.

Think of categories of things through the alphabet: for example : countries beginning with A, with B, with C etc.

Try other subjects: whatever interests you. Just think out of your normal box; it makes life much more interesting.

If you choose a dull subject this is a good way to bore yourself to sleep.

Remember to do some of these suggestions, but if you get bored of them make up your own that you find more interesting.

Get into the habit of thinking in as many different ways as possible.

Waste Some Time.

Once Mr. Daddy Long-Legs,
Dressed in brown and grey,
Walked about upon the sands
Upon a summer's day;
And there among the pebbles,
When the wind was rather cold,
He met with Mr. Floppy Fly,
All dressed in blue and gold.
As it was too soon to dine,
They drank some periwinkle-wine,
And played an hour or two, or more,
At battle cock and shuttledore.

Edward Lear

Decisions.

Decide on a meal you can cook. Then cook it. You may have to shop somewhere different.

What will you do tomorrow that is different from today?

What was the best decision you've ever made?

How About a Bit of Romance?
Even a holiday? Real or imagined.

Like the owl and the pussycat.

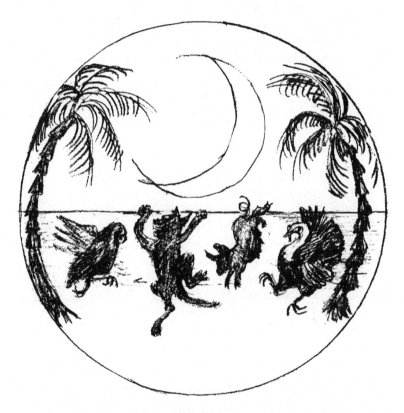

The Owl and the Pussy-Cat went to sea
In a beautiful pea-green boat,
They took some honey, and plenty of money,
Wrapped up in a five pound note.
The Owl looked up at the stars above,
And sang to a small guitar
"O lovely Pussy! O Pussy, my love,
"What a beautiful Pussy you are,
"You are,
"You are!
"What a beautiful Pussy you are!"

Pussy said to the Owl, "You elegant fowl!
"How charmingly sweet you sing!
"O let us be married! Too long have we tarried:
"But what shall we do for a ring?"
They sailed away for a year and a day,
To the land where the Bong-tree grows,
And there in the wood a Piggy-wig stood,
With a ring in the end of his nose,
His nose,
His nose,
With a ring in the end of his nose.

"Dear Pig, are you willing to sell for one shilling
"Your ring?" Said the Piggy, "I will".
So they took it away and were married next day
By the Turkey who lived on the hill.
They dined on mince, and slices of quince,
Which they ate with a runcible spoon;
And hand in hand, on the edge of the sand,
They danced by the light of the moon,
The moon,
The moon,
They danced by the light of the moon.

Enjoy making your brain work (and not just at work).

But: BEWARE!

Much learning doth make thee mad.

The Acts of The Apostles

Index

ISBN 142510658-7

9 781425 106584

Printed in Great Britain
by Amazon

25803111R00056